3-DAY DIET PLAN FOR WEIGHTLOSS

Delicious Recipes for a Healthy and Balanced Lifestyle

Contents

Understanding Weight Loss

Weight loss is a complex process that involves both physical and mental aspects. Understanding how it works and how to achieve it can help you make the most of your efforts.

When it comes to weight loss, it's important to remember that a calorie deficit is the key. A calorie deficit occurs when you take in fewer calories than you burn. This forces your body to use stored fat for energy, leading to weight loss. To achieve a calorie deficit, you must either reduce your calorie intake, increase your physical activity, or both.

Exercise is an important part of any weight loss program. Regular physical activity helps burn calories and increases your overall health. It's important to choose activities that you enjoy, so you'll be more likely to stick with them. Examples of physical activities include walking, running, swimming, and strength training.

In addition to exercise, nutrition plays a critical role in weight loss. Eating nutritious foods can help you stay on track and maintain a healthy weight. Eating a balanced diet and controlling portion sizes can help you maintain a healthy body weight. Eating healthy foods such as fruits, vegetables, whole grains, lean proteins, and healthy fats is important. Limiting your intake of processed and high-calorie foods is also important.

Another important factor when it comes to weight loss is mental health. Managing stress levels and getting enough sleep can play a big role in your success. Stress can increase cortisol levels, which can cause you to overeat and gain weight. Reducing stress and getting adequate sleep can help you stay on track with your weight loss goals.

Finally, setting realistic goals is essential for success. Aiming for too much too soon can lead to frustration and ultimately, failure. Instead, set realistic goals that you can achieve, such as drinking more water, eating more vegetables, or exercising 3 times a week.

Overall, weight loss is a complex process that involves both physical and mental aspects. Understanding how it works and how to achieve it can help you make the most of your efforts. Eating a balanced diet, exercising regularly, and managing stress levels are all important components of a successful weight loss

program.

What Causes Weight Gain?

Weight gain is a complex and multi-faceted issue. There are many factors that can contribute to weight gain, including lifestyle choices, genetics, and even certain medical conditions. Understanding the causes of weight gain can help you better manage your weight and make healthier lifestyle choices.

One of the most common causes of weight gain is eating too much and not getting enough physical activity. Eating too many unhealthy foods, such as those high in sugar, fat, and calories, can lead to weight gain. Additionally, not getting enough physical activity can also contribute to weight gain. This can be especially true if you tend to sit for long periods of time.

Genetics can also play a role in weight gain. Some people are genetically predisposed to gaining weight more easily than others. Additionally, certain medical conditions can be linked to weight gain. These conditions can include hypothyroidism, Cushing's syndrome, and polycystic ovarian syndrome.

Stress can also lead to weight gain. Stress is linked to changes in hormones that can lead to changes in appetite and cravings for unhealthy foods. Additionally, stress can lead to changes in eating habits, such as eating too much or too often.

Finally, certain medications can be linked to weight gain. These medications can include some antidepressants, steroids, and diabetes medications. Before beginning any medication, it is important to speak to your physician about any potential side effects, including weight gain.

Weight gain is a complicated issue with many potential causes. By understanding the different causes of weight gain, you can make healthier lifestyle choices and better manage your weight. Additionally, if you think that you may be suffering from a medical condition that is contributing to your weight gain, it is important to speak to your physician to get the appropriate treatment.

The Benefits of Weight Loss

Weight loss can be one of the most rewarding and beneficial changes you can make in your life. It can lead to improved physical and mental health, as well as a greater sense of self-confidence and self-esteem. Here are some of the top benefits of weight loss.

1. Improved Physical Health: Weight loss can lead to improved physical health and reduce the risk of developing certain diseases, such as

diabetes, heart disease, and some forms of cancer. It can also help improve blood pressure and cholesterol levels, which can reduce the risk of stroke and other cardiovascular issues.

2. Improved Mental Health: Weight loss can also lead to improved mental health. It can help reduce stress and anxiety, and can even help with depression. Studies have also found that weight loss can improve self-esteem and body image, which can

lead to improved mental health overall.

3. Increased Energy Levels: Losing weight can lead to increased energy levels. This can help you feel more alert and able to handle physical and mental tasks more effectively. It can also make it easier to get through a tough day at work or to tackle a tough workout.

4. Improved Mobility: Weight loss can also lead to improved mobility. This

can make it easier to do everyday tasks, such as carrying groceries or climbing stairs. It can also make it easier to participate in activities that require more physical activity, such as running, biking, or swimming.

5. Reduced Risk of Injury: Weight loss can help reduce the risk of injury, as it can make it easier to move around and perform everyday tasks without strain or discomfort. It can also help reduce the risk of developing osteoarthritis, as the extra weight can put extra strain

on the joints and lead to wear and tear on the cartilage.

These are just a few of the many benefits of weight loss. If you're looking to make a lifestyle change that will improve your overall health and wellbeing, then weight loss should be at the top of your list. So, if you're ready to make a change, get started today and start seeing the rewards of weight loss.

Setting Realistic weight loss Goals

When it comes to weight loss, setting realistic goals is key to achieving success. Unattainable goals can lead to frustration and feelings of failure, so it's important to be honest with yourself and set realistic expectations.

Start by asking yourself a few questions: What is a reasonable amount of time to lose the weight? What changes can you make to your lifestyle and diet to help you reach your goal?

It's important to set a timeline for your weight loss goals. A month or two is often a realistic timeframe to shed a few pounds. However, if you have a significant amount of weight to lose, it's important to remember that it will take time. Setting a timeline that is too short can lead to frustration and disappointment.

It's also important to create a plan for how you will reach your goals. This could include making changes to your diet, such as reducing your calorie intake or eliminating processed foods. You may also want to set a goal to increase your physical activity, such as walking for 30 minutes every day.

In addition to diet and exercise, it is also important to take into account other factors such as stress, sleep, and mental health. All of these things can affect your ability to reach your goals.

Finally, it's important to remember that weight loss is not a linear process. You may have days where you don't seem to make progress, and that's okay. Stay motivated by celebrating the small successes and keeping your eye on the long-term goal.

Setting realistic weight loss goals can help you stay motivated and on track. Be honest with yourself and take into account all the factors that may affect your progress. With a plan and the right attitude, you can achieve your

goals.

Choosing the Right Diet for weight loss

When it comes to losing weight, one of the most important decisions you will make is choosing the right diet. With so many diets on the market, it can be difficult to decide which one is best for you. However, understanding the basics of how to pick the right diet can help you make an informed decision and ensure that you are successful in your weight loss journey.

First and foremost, it's important to make sure that the diet you choose is safe and healthy. Many fad diets promise quick and easy results, but they are often unhealthy and can even be dangerous. It's important to educate yourself on the science behind any diet you're considering and make sure that it is balanced and nutritious.

Second, consider your lifestyle. While some diets may be effective, they may not be practical for your lifestyle. If you have a busy job or a family, it can be difficult to commit to the strict schedule that some diets require. Consider your schedule and make sure that the diet you choose fits into it.

Third, consider your goals. Different diets work for different people. For some, the goal may be to lose weight quickly, while others may be focused on developing healthier habits that can be maintained over time. Decide what your goals are and find a diet that will help you achieve them.

Finally, be sure to seek professional help. While it's possible to choose a diet on your own, it's always a good idea to consult with a doctor or nutritionist who can assess your individual needs and recommend a diet that is right for you.

Choosing the right diet can be a daunting task, but with the right information and support, you can find the diet that best suits your lifestyle and goals. By understanding the basics of how to pick the right diet and seeking professional help, you can

ensure that you are successful in your

weight loss journey.

Achieving and maintaining a healthy weight is essential to good health, and it can be difficult to do without a plan. Building a healthy eating plan for weight loss requires a commitment to making healthier eating choices more often and incorporating physical activity into your daily routine. Fortunately, it doesn't need to be complicated or expensive. With some simple changes, you can create a plan that will help you lose weight and keep it off for the long term.

The first step to building a healthy eating plan for weight loss is to assess your current eating habits and determine what needs to change. Start by keeping a food journal for a few days or a week. This will help you identify patterns of eating that may be contributing to your weight gain. Then, you should focus on making small changes that you can stick with for the long term. This could include cutting down portion sizes, adding more fruits and vegetables to your meals, reducing your intake of unhealthy fats and sugars, and increasing your consumption of whole grains and lean proteins.

In addition, it's important to create a meal plan that is balanced and nutritious. This means eating foods from all of the major food groups in appropriate portions. Aim to include a variety of fruits, vegetables, whole grains, lean proteins, and healthy fats in your meals and snacks. Eating a balanced diet will ensure that you get all the essential nutrients your body needs.

When creating a healthy eating plan for weight loss, it's also important to include physical activity. Physical activity helps burn calories and increases metabolism, which can help speed up weight loss. Aim to get 30 minutes of moderate physical activity most days of the week. This could include walking, jogging, biking, swimming, or any other form of physical activity that you enjoy.

Finally, it's important to stay motivated and keep track of your progress. Make sure to celebrate your successes and keep at it even when it gets tough. Consider setting realistic goals and rewarding yourself when you reach them.

Creating a healthy eating plan for weight loss can be a challenge, but it is possible. With some planning and dedication, you can develop a plan that will help you lose weight and keep it off for the long term.

The 3-Day Diet Plan: Everything You Need To Know

Do you want to lose weight quickly for an upcoming event or to jump-start your weight loss? Are you uncomfortable with your excess weight? Then the best way to lose weight is to follow a very low-calorie diet for three days every two weeks. During this 3-day diet, you do not have to go on a fast or starve yourself. You will eat nutritious foods but cut back on the unnecessary calories. You will also exercise on the non-diet days to help you mobilize the fat and get a toned body. But mind you, to avoid health issues it is advisable not to follow this diet plan continuously for more than two weeks. In this article, I will discuss the 3-day diet plan, foods to eat and avoid, non-diet days exercise plan, and much more. So hang in there and let me show you the easiest way to lose weight. Shall we begin?

How the 3-Day Diet Plan Works

The 3-day diet works by restricting the calorie consumption to less than 1200 per day for three days a week. You will go back to normal diet for the rest of the four days of the week without exceeding a limit of consuming 500 calories extra. For example, if you have 1000 calories on the diet days, you will not consume more than 1500 calories per day on non-diet days. This varied calorie intake will prevent your body's metabolism from plateauing and help you burn the calories and lose weight quickly. Always follow the 3-day diet plan for two weeks and then take a break for one week before resuming this diet plan. Let's find out what you should eat for three days of your very low-calorie diet plan.

The 3-Day Diet Plan

Day 1 (1200 calories)

Meals   What To Eat

Early Morning (7:45 – 8:30 a.m)1 cup fenugreek seeds soaked water

Breakfast (9:15-9:45 a.m) Options:

•   Oatmeal (40 g oats + 150 ml low fat milk+ 15 g nuts mixture + any fruit of choice 1 serving)

•   2 egg whites + 1 multigrain toast + 1 fresh whole fruit/ Fruit juice with pulp (No sweetener)

Lunch   (12:00   –   12:30   p.m) Options:

•   Grilled fish in asparagus and tomato sauce

•   Tuna/vegetable sandwich (Use whole wheat or multigrain bread)

Evening Snack (4:00 p.m) Options:

- Bowl of fruits

- ½ cup baby carrots

Dinner (7:00 – 7:30 p.m) Options:

- Garlic bread (1pc) and chicken stewed in Italian herbs

- Smoked turkey cakes and 1 pita bread with lots of sliced cucumber, tomato, and onion.

Why This Works

Fenugreek soaked water helps to boost your metabolism and prevents constipation. Oats are full of fiber, which helps prevent fat absorption and helps to mobilize fat. Eggs are an excellent source of protein, and multigrain bread is high in fiber content. Fresh fruit juice is rich in fiber, and fruit sugar will keep your hunger pangs at bay for longer.. Have a delicious but light lunch rich in protein, fiber, and complex carbs. Choose grilled fish or a sandwich to satiate your taste buds. Have a substantial portion of complex carbs and fiber in the form of fruits or crunchy vegetable for a healthy evening snack. Spice up your dinner by having garlic bread (multigrain) and chicken stew, which is rich in protein and other nutrients. If you do not want to have chicken, opt for turkey, also a rich source of protein. Have cucumber, tomato, and onion to balance your high-protein meal with complex carbs and dietary fiber.

Substitutes

Fenugreek seeds – Fennel seeds

Oatmeal – Quinoa

Scrambled eggs – Boiled eggs

Multigrain bread – wheat or gluten-free bread

Fresh fruit juice – 1/2 cup fruit

Grilled fish – Baked or smoked fish

Asparagus – Spinach

Tomato – Finely diced cucumber

Tuna sandwich – Chicken sandwich

Vegetable sandwich – mushroom sandwich

Fruits – 1 cup fresh fruit juice

Baby carrots – 1 cup large cubes of cucumber

Garlic bread – Wheat flatbread

Chicken stew – Grilled chicken with glaze

Smoked turkey – Smoked salmon or crab

Pita bread – multigrain bread or flatbread

Cucumber – Carrot

Tomato – Red bell pepper

Onion – Chive

How You Will Feel By The End Of Day 1

Day 1 would be tough. You will feel hungry and crave for junk food. But what you will gain by not munching on junk is greater and more important to you right now. Control your hunger pangs by drinking water or green tea.

Day 2 (1000 calories)

Meals   What To Eat

Early Morning (7:45 – 8:30 a.m)1 glass warm water with the juice of half a lime

Breakfast (9:15-9:45 a.m) Options:

Quinoa + 1 cup green tea

Egg frittata + 1 cup green tea

Lunch (12:00 – 12:30 p.m) Options:

- Sauteed green beans, peas, carrots, and mushroom + ½ cup fat-free yogurt

- Grilled chicken breast (2 oz) with broccoli, spinach, and carrots + 1 cup low-fat buttermilk

Evening Snack (4:00 p.m) 1 cup black coffee

Dinner (7:00 – 7:30 p.m) Options:

- Chicken/ vegetable soup + ½ cup low-fat vanilla ice cream

- Boiled chickpeas salad + ½ cup low-fat vanilla ice cream

Why This Works

Lime juice works by helping to mobilize the fat and flushing out toxins. Quinoa or egg frittata with a cup of green tea will help keep you full and suppress your appetite. Have a nutritious and delicious lunch with sauteed veggies and mushroom or grilled chicken and veggies. Low-fat yogurt or buttermilk will ensure better digestion, which, in turn, will lead to better metabolism. Black coffee is a great appetite suppressant and also improves alertness and concentration. Have a delicious dinner loaded with protein sources such as chicken or boiled chickpeas. Half a cup of vanilla ice cream will appease your taste buds.

Substitutes

Lime – Lemon or apple cider vinegar

Quinoa – Oats

Egg frittata – Spanish omelet or boiled eggs

Green tea – Oolong tea or black coffee

Green beans – Asparagus

Peas – Endive

Carrot – Yellow bell pepper

Mushroom – Baby corn

Fat-free yogurt – 1 cup fresh ginger, fennel seed, and lime juice

Chicken breast – Salmon / mushroom

Broccoli – Cauliflower

Spinach – Celery

Carrots – Tomato

Buttermilk – 1 cup watermelon juice

Black coffee – green tea or oolong tea

Chicken / Vegetable soup – Lentil / mushroom soup

Boiled chickpea salad – Bengal gram salad or chicken salad

Vanilla ice cream – Frozen yogurt

How You Will Feel By The End Of Day 2

By the end of day 2, you will be surprised to find out that you survived two days without munching on junk food! This will keep your spirits high, and you will be ready for day 3 more than ever.

Day 3 (800 calories)

Meals   What To Eat

Early Morning (7:45 – 8:30 a.m)1 cup water with 1 teaspoon apple cider vinegar

Breakfast (9:15-9:45 a.m) Options:

•   2 boiled egg whites + 1 cup musk melon and pomegranate smoothie

- ½ cup vegetable semolina (20 g) + ½ cup fat-free milk

Lunch (12:00 – 12:30 p.m) Options:

- Chicken salad with fat-free yogurt, olive oil, salt, and pepper dressing

- Grilled tuna with collard greens and cherry tomatoes

Evening Snack (4:00 p.m) 1 cup green tea

Dinner (7:00 – 7:30 p.m) Options:

- Oven baked chicken stuffed bell pepper

- Chicken or mushroom soup with Asian herbs and seasoning

Why This Works

Apple cider vinegar helps in weight loss and regulates blood pressure. Have a large protein rich breakfast to feed your brain and muscles so that you can stay active. If you want to have salad for lunch, opt for a low-fat dressing. Grilled tuna will keep your taste buds alive and provide your body an extra dose of protein. Green tea is best for losing weight and suppressing appetite. Make your boring dinner interesting by adding Mexican or Asian touch while keeping it nutritious and simple. This will help you stay nourished throughout the day while maintaining the calorie count.

Substitutes

Apple cider vinegar – Lemon juice

Boiled egg whites – Egg white omelet

Muskmelon – Watermelon

Pomegranate – Cherries

Semolina – Quinoa

Milk – Soy milk

Chicken salad – Tuna or veggie salad

Yogurt – Sour cream

Olive oil – Flax seed oil

Tuna – Basa

Collard greens – Spinach

Cherry tomato – Summer squash

Green tea – Oolong tea or black coffee

Chicken – Mushroom or chickpeas

Bell pepper – Squash

Chicken or mushroom soup – Grilled

veggies or vegetable soup

How You Will Feel By The End Of Day 3

By the end of day 3, you would have lost a lot of water weight. This means you would look slimmer and feel less bloated. Your body would be ready to mobilize the fat, and that is exactly what exercising would help to achieve. So, though you have lost water weight, to actually lose fat you have to exercise on the non-diet days. Here is an exercise plan for Days 4 – 7.

Exercise Plan For Non-Diet Days (Day 4 – Day 7)

Warm-up (10 min)

- Move your head side to side 10 times.

- Move your head up and down as if you are nodding, 10 times.

- Neck rotations (clockwise and anti-clockwise) – 1 set of 10 reps

- Shoulder rotations (clockwise and anti-clockwise) – 1 set of 10 reps

- Full arm rotation (clockwise and anti-clockwise) – 1 set of 10 reps

- Wrist rotation (clockwise and anti-clockwise) – 1 set of 10 reps

- Waist rotation (clockwise and anti-clockwise) – 1 set of 10 reps

- Ankle rotation (clockwise and anti-clockwise) – 1 set of 10 reps

- Standing side crunches (left and right)- 1 set of 10 reps

- Touch toes – 1 set of 5 reps

Days Time What You Should Do

Day 4   15 min   Spot jogging + Side lunges + Jumping jacks +

Forward lunges + Scissor kicks + Push-ups + Stretch

Day 5   25 min   Brisk walking / intermittent jogging + Forward jumping lunges + Squat + Bicep curls + Tricep dips + Forward plank + Side plank + Crunches + Meditation

Day 6   40 min   Rope jumping + Forward lunges with weight + Push-ups + Crunches + Mountain climbers + Burpees + Horizontal outward kicks + scissor kicks + Stretch

Day 7   50 min   Intermittent walking and jogging + Surya Namaskar+ Meditation

Make sure not to workout rigorously from Day 1 – Day 3 (diet days) as you will be on a very low-calorie diet and your body may not have the required energy. However, you may do light stretching exercises on your diet days.

How You Will Feel By The End Of Day 7

You will be both surprised and thrilled with your progress. The first 3 days of the diet will help you lose water weight and the last 4 days of the week will help you mobilize the fat. This will help you to lose weight quicker and more effectively. You will look slimmer and working out regularly will help you stay active and focussed. It will also improve memory and reflex, and remove all negative thoughts from your mind.

Should You Repeat The 3-Day Diet?

Yes, you can go on the 3-day diet again in the second week. The second week may not feel challenging enough, but you should stick to the diet plan to get optimum results.

Should You Continue The 3-Day Diet Beyond The Second Week?

No. This diet plan may work well for you, but it is advisable not to continue with this diet beyond the second week. You can be on a low-calorie diet and exercise to keep your body from gaining the weight back. You can follow the 3-day diet plan after taking a week's break. You should also talk to your dietician or doctor before deciding to be on this diet indefinitely.

Now, it is not easy to consume less and suppress your appetite. We have some tricks on how to suppress appetite and here is what we recommend you to do when you are on the 3-day diet plan.

How Can You Reduce Your Appetite?

Feeling starved is a phenomenon that is a part of almost every diet due to the restrictions placed on certain foods. Thus, decreasing the appetite makes the diet relatively easier to follow. A limited portion of food is consumed during the 3-day diet, and so these tips can be followed to decrease the appetite and trigger weight loss.

• Drinking water: Drinking water throughout the day will quench your hunger to a great extent. Besides, research has proved that water consumption accelerates the rate at which calories are burnt. Moreover, drinking lime/lemon water is particularly helpful in losing weight. At least 8 glasses of fluids every day are recommended for better results.

•	Getting enough sleep: Those who do not get enough sleep tend to feel more hungry and thus have a greater appetite. This is because the body hormones go into a direction that leads to weight gain. Hence, the importance of sleep cannot be undermined.

•	Drink Green Tea: Green tea helps to suppress appetite and the best time to consume it is 30 minutes before a meal. Since green tea has zero calories, you can consume it in between the meals. But make sure not to drink more than 3 cups of green tea per day.

The 3-day diet also has the following benefits:

3-Day Diet Benefits

- It is effective when it comes to rapid weight loss (about 10 pounds in 3 days).

- It is cheap as the foods like coffee, tuna, and vegetables are affordable.

- It is simple and easy to follow as ingredients are easily available, and the meals are simple and can be quickly prepared.

- Weight loss leads to several cardiovascular benefits such as reduced blood pressure and a decrease in bad LDL cholesterol.

- No side effects, whatsoever, are associated with this diet. However, those who have health issues should consult their physician before following it.

So, the bottom line is the 3-day diet plan appears like an ideal way to lose weight. But it also helps to know the drawbacks before starting it.

3-Day Diet Drawbacks

•	The 3-day diet is considered as a fad diet. Though it is effective for weight loss, much of it is lean muscle mass or water weight is quickly regained once you start eating normally.

•	This diet can cause electrolyte imbalance which disrupts the normal heart rhythm leading to massive loss of water weight and muscle cramping. This upsets the balance of certain minerals in the body like potassium which may interfere with the function of your heart with fatal consequences.

•   Though the weight loss leads to cardiovascular benefits, gaining and losing weight on a continuous basis can stress the heart.

•   Following this diet on a regular basis can cause nutrient deficiencies, long-term weight gain, a weakened immune system, and heart problems. It is low in iron and calcium. Deficiency of iron can cause anemia, and lack of calcium can weaken the bones.

- This diet is potentially dangerous for those with diabetes.

- You have to compromise your taste buds as there are no exotic ingredients, frozen meals or powdered shakes. Moreover, it eliminates snacks from the menu altogether.

- This diet is not suitable for children and teens because a growing child requires adequate calories and nutrition for development and this diet is lacking in both. Moreover, it can cause potential eating disorders.

So, the 3-day diet plan is not for those looking for a long-term weight loss diet plan. But you can follow the 3-day diet plan to lose weight quickly and effectively for a special occasion. Follow the diet chart and workout plan, and you can see results in the first week. Begin today and get ready to wow everyone! Take care.

Conclusion

The 3-day diet plan is not for those looking for a long-term weight loss diet plan. Calorie counting and portion control are the golden rules to stay fit and healthy without compromising on nutrients. Eat slowly, chew well, include good bioavailable proteins in your diet and keep yourself hydrated to keep your metabolism at its best.

The Promise

These days, when even instant cereal isn't fast enough, we want weight loss now, not later. And who could argue with dropping the weight of a large laptop in just one long weekend? The 3 Day Diet promises exactly that.

If you've been struggling to budge the scale and you're tempted to try it, here are the details you need to know.

The diet, aimed at people wanting to lose a lot of weight, claims you'll drop up to 10 pounds if you follow it for three days.

The menu consists of three breakfasts, lunches, and "dinners" -- if you consider a cup of tuna fish or two hot dogs, plus fruit and vegetable sides, dinner.

A website that markets the diet claims it's "chemically and enzyme balanced," though this statement isn't explained or supported.

One thing is clear: You won't be eating much. On Day 1, you get just 870 calories. Days 2 and 3 aren't much different.

What You Can Eat and What You Can't

For three days, you'll eat extremely basic meals made with foods you may already have in your kitchen.

For example, breakfast on Day 1 is black coffee or water, half a grapefruit, and a slice of toast with 2 tablespoons of peanut butter. Lunch is half a cup of tuna, another slice of toast, and another cup of black coffee (or tea or water).

If you're looking for variety or foodie thrills, you won't find them here.

Lunch on Day 2, for instance, is nothing but a cup of cottage cheese, one hard boiled egg, and some saltine crackers. Sauces, dressings, and even spices are off the list. If you have a sweet tooth, though, you'll be happy to find vanilla ice cream on the menu each day.

Level of Effort: Low

The biggest effort you'll make on the diet may be stopping yourself from reaching for more food.

Limitations: The menu is what it is, with no room for varied palates or eating preferences, though some web sites say you can swap tuna for cottage cheese and vice versa.

Cooking and shopping: This diet is about as low-effort as it gets, short of having meals delivered to your door. Just about the only cooking involved is steaming the vegetables, unless you choose to eat them raw (either is an option).

Packaged foods or meals? No.

In-person meetings? No.

Exercise: It's frowned on because, as one website puts it, "you will not be feeling very energetic" while you're on this diet.

Does It Allow for Dietary Restrictions or Preferences?

Vegetarians and vegans: This menu is not for vegetarians or vegans. It's not low-salt, low-carb, or low-fat, either -- just low-calorie.

Gluten-free: This diet includes toast and crackers, which traditionally include gluten in the wheat. You could buy gluten-free versions if you chose to, but going gluten-free is not a feature of this diet.

What Else You Should Know

This diet was most likely not developed by nutrition experts. One web site that offers the diet includes this warning: "Neither the staff nor management of 3 Day Diets are experienced, licensed, or knowledgeable to judge or recommend the validity or safety of this diet. We do not necessarily endorse this diet and recommend that before trying this or any other diet to consult a physician or licensed medical practitioner. Use at your own risk."

When judging any diet, including this one, keep in mind two key pieces of advice from the Academy of Nutrition and Dietetics: First, if a diet sounds too good to be true, it probably is. Second, if you can't see yourself following the diet for the rest of your life, it's not for you.

Costs: None beyond your shopping.

Support: None. This is a diet you do on your own.

What Dr. Melinda Ratini Says:

Does It Work?

You will likely lose weight on any diet if you eat less than 910 calories a day. But losing 10 pounds in 3 days is both unlikely and unhealthy. To lose just 1 pound of body fat, you need to reduce your daily calories by about 500 a day for a whole week. That's giving up 3,500 calories over the course of 7 days. To lose 10 pounds in 3 days would mean decreasing your calorie intake by 35,000 calories in just 3 days! The Academy of Nutrition and Dietetics recommends a slow and steady weight loss of no more than 1/2 to 1 pound a week. Otherwise you are losing muscle and water, as well as weakening your bones. You also are much more likely to gain it all back.

Is It Good for Certain Conditions?

The 3 Day Diet is low calorie, but it certainly is not low-fat, low-salt, or low cholesterol, so it is not a healthy option for most people with certain medical conditions such as diabetes, hypertension, heart disease, and high cholesterol. If you are overweight, weight loss is key to managing these conditions. But it should be a healthy and sustainable weight loss that includes healthy nutrition and exercise.

The Final Word

The 3 Day Diet is a very low-calorie diet that uses simple foods that are low cost and easy to find and prepare. A short-term weight loss is likely. But that is where the good news ends.

During the 3 days of the diet, balanced nutrition is lacking. Some of the foods that are recommended are high in salt and fat and would not be appropriate for people with certain medical problems like heart disease, high blood pressure, diabetes, or high cholesterol. You may not be getting enough vitamins, minerals, and fiber while you are on the diet. If you are taking medicine for your diabetes and want to try the 3-day diet, it's important to talk with your doctor first about how to adjust your medicine.

Physical activity is an important part of a healthy lifestyle and helps prevent and treat heart disease and diabetes. But the 3 Day Diet does not address this at all. Nor does it teach you how to make changes in your diet that will allow for a lifetime of healthy eating.

Finally, such a restrictive diet takes the enjoyment out of eating. During the 3 days a week that you are following the plan, eating out or with others could be very tough. Also, boring diets are very hard to maintain. The temptation to overeat on the other 4 days of the week when you are not dieting will likely be high.

Remember, when it comes to weight loss, slow and steady really does win the race.

www.ingramcontent.com/pod-product-compliance
Lightning Source LLC
Chambersburg PA
CBHW061555250726
48657CB00021B/1797